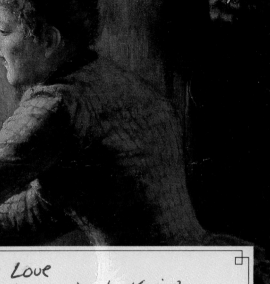

Love
From: Uncle Kevin
Aunty Lano
Allan, Rebecca.
+ Justin
xo xo xo xo

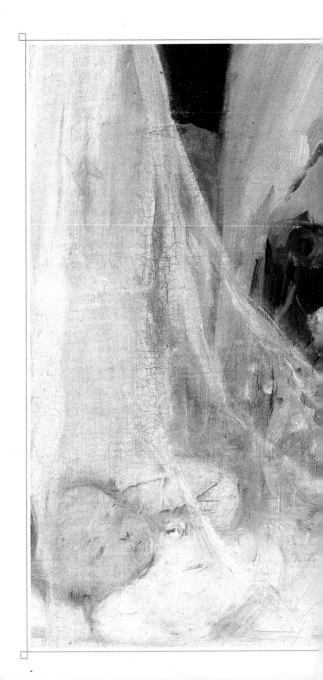

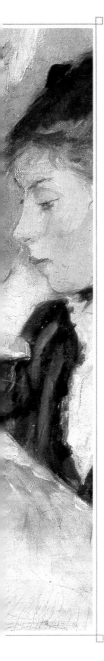

There is nothing on earth like the moment of seeing one's first baby. Men scale other heights, but there is no height like this simple one, occurring continuously throughout all the ages in musty bedrooms, in palaces, in caves and desert places. I looked at this rolled-up bundle...and knew again I had not created her. She was herself apart from me. She had her own life to lead, her own destiny to accomplish; she just came past me to this earth. My job was to get her to adulthood and then push her off.

KATHERINE TREVELYAN.
from *Through Mine Own Eyes*

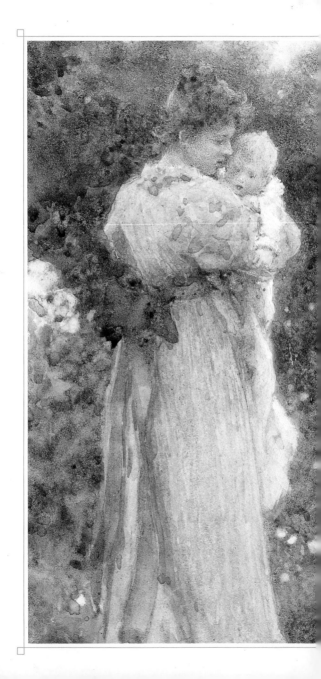

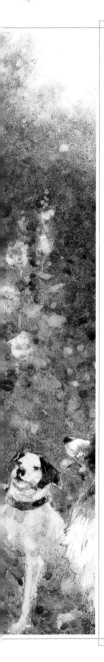

Then they handed her to me, stiff and howling, and I held her for the first time and kissed her, and she went still and quiet as though by instinctive guile, and I was utterly enslaved by her flattery of my powers.

LAURIE LEE. b.1914.
from *The Firstborn*

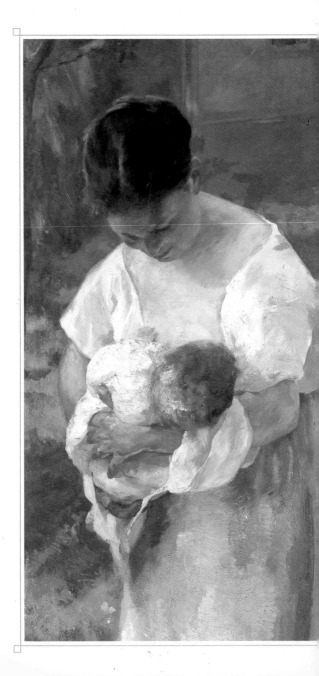

The parents exist to teach
the child, but also they
must learn what the child
has to teach them; and the
child has a very great deal
to teach them.

ARNOLD BENNETT (1867-1931)

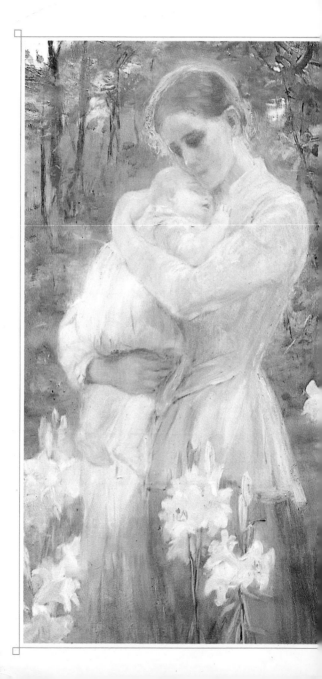

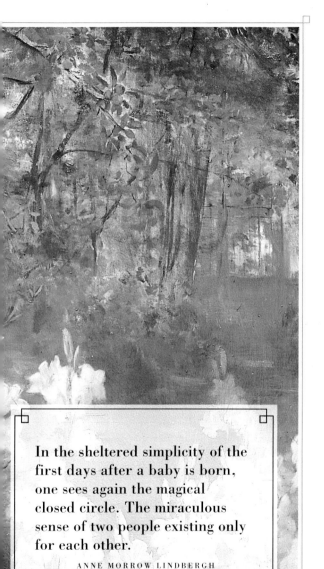

In the sheltered simplicity of the
first days after a baby is born,
one sees again the magical
closed circle. The miraculous
sense of two people existing only
for each other.

ANNE MORROW LINDBERGH

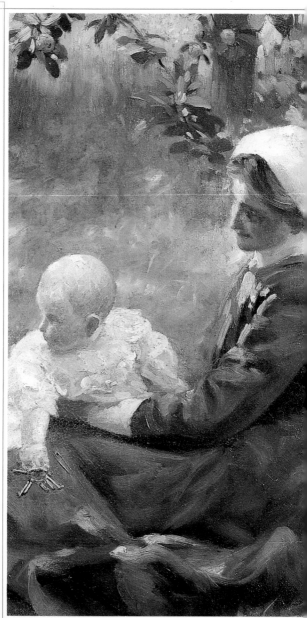

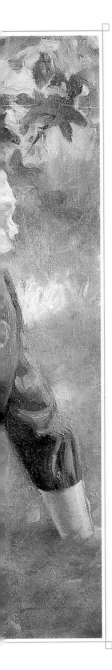

In every work the beginning
is the most important part,
especially in dealing with
anything young and tender.

SOCRATES (469-399 B.C.)

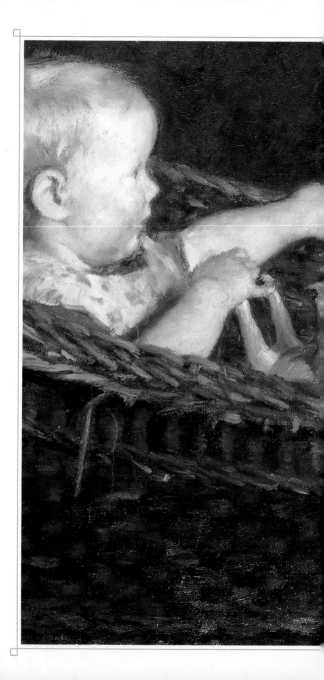

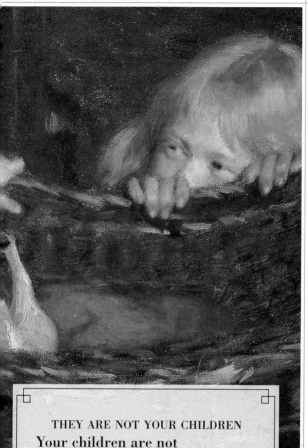

**THEY ARE NOT YOUR CHILDREN**
Your children are not
your children.
They are the sons and
daughters of Life's longing
for itself.

KAHLIL GIBRAN (1883-1931),
from *The Prophet*

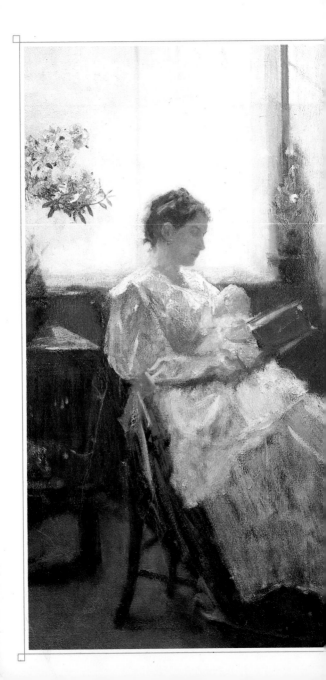

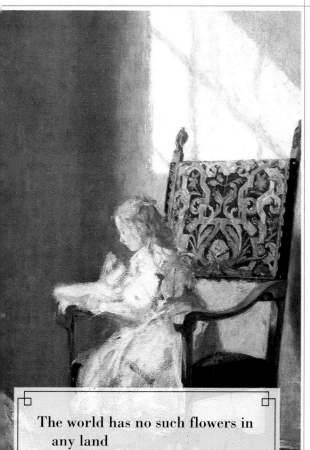

The world has no such flowers in
    any land
And no such pearl in any gulf the
    sea
As any babe on any mother's
    knee.

ALGERNON CHARLES SWINBURNE
(1897-1909), from *Pelagius*

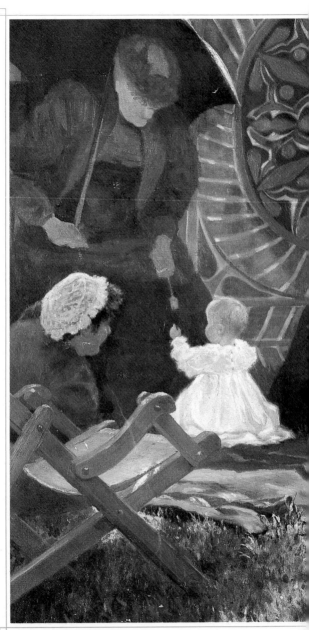

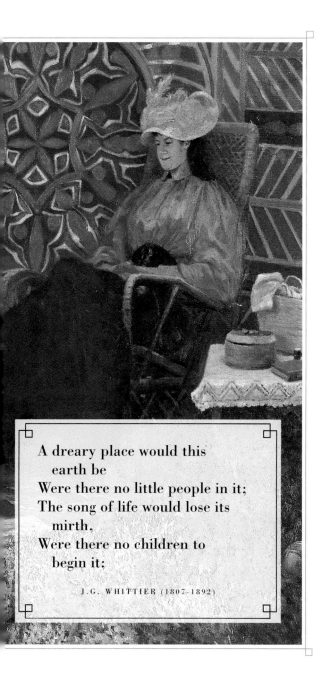

A dreary place would this
  earth be
Were there no little people in it;
The song of life would lose its
  mirth,
Were there no children to
  begin it;

J.G. WHITTIER (1807-1892)

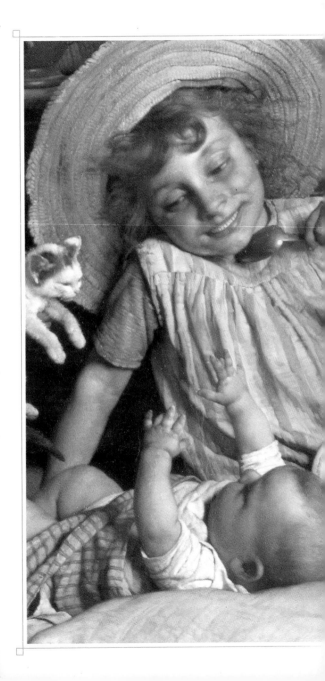

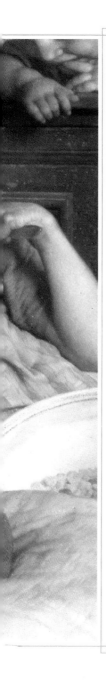

The baby has learned to smile, and her smiles burst forth like holiday sparklers, lighting our hearts. Joy fills the room.

At what are we smiling? We don't know, and we don't care. We are communicating with one another in happiness, and the smiles are the outward display of our delight and our love.

JOAN LOWERY NIXON,
from *The Grandmother's Book*

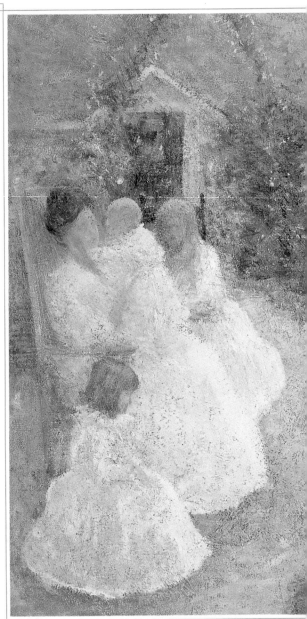

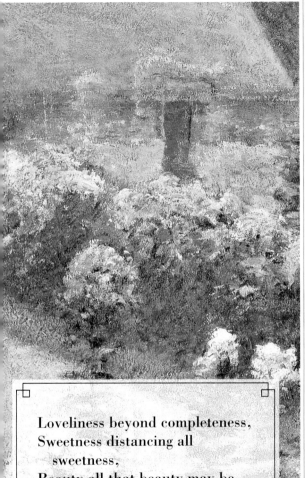

Loveliness beyond completeness,
Sweetness distancing all
    sweetness,
Beauty all that beauty may be –
That's May Bennett, that's
    my baby.

WILLIAM COX BENNETT

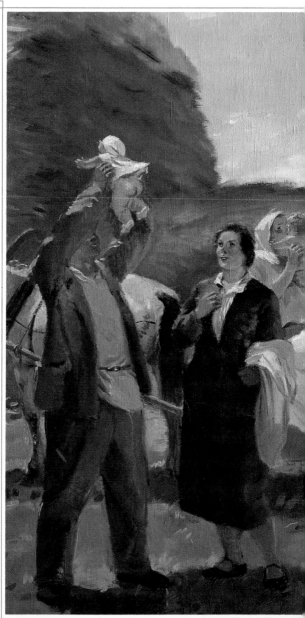

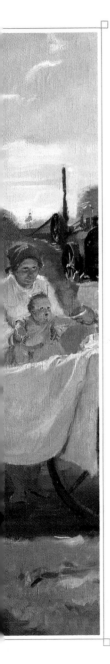

Thou, straggler into loving
arms,
Young climber-up of knees,
When I forget thy thousand
ways
Then life and all shall
cease.

MARY LAMB